EAT TO BEAT POTS SYNDROME

Optimal Nutrition For Postural Orthostatic Tachycardia Syndrome: A POTS-Friendly Diet That Can Alter Your Health

DR. LONDYN DELANEY

Copyright © 2024 By Dr. Londyn Delaney

All Rights Reserved...

Table of Contents

Introductory 6
CHAPTER ONE 9
  Types Of POTS 9
  Symptoms And Diagnosis 13
CHAPTER TWO 19
  Causes And Risk Factors 19
  Pathophysiology Of POTS 24
CHAPTER THREE 31
  How Diet Affects POTS Symptoms & Nutritional Needs Of POTS Patients 31
  Creating A POTS-Friendly Meal Plan 37
CHAPTER FOUR 45
  Grocery Shopping Tips 45
  Meal Prep And Cooking Tips 51
CHAPTER FIVE 58
  Food Sensitivities And Allergies 58
  Gluten-Free And Dairy-Free Options 64
CHAPTER SIX 72
  Vegetarian And Vegan Diets 72

- Energizing Smoothies Recipes For Breakfast 81
- High-Protein Breakfast Bowls Recipes . 88
- Salt-Rich Breakfast Ideas Recipes 96

CHAPTER SEVEN 104
- Light And Nourishing Salads Recipes For Lunch 104
- Protein-Packed Sandwiches And Wraps Recipes 113
- Electrolyte-Rich Soups Recipes 120

CHAPTER EIGHT 131
- Balanced And Satisfying Main Courses Recipes For Dinner 131
- Easy And Quick Dinner Ideas Recipes . 142
- Slow Cooker And One-Pot Meals Recipes 151

CHAPTER NINE 162
- Healthy Snack Options Recipes 162
- Hydrating Beverages Recipes 168
- Salt-Rich Snacks Recipes 174

CHAPTER TEN 182

Exercise And Physical Activity 182

Managing Stress And Sleep 189

CHAPTER ELEVEN 197

Monitoring And Adjusting Your Diet .. 197

Conclusion 204

THE END 208

Introductory

When a person gets up from a seated or laying posture, they may experience a set of symptoms known as Postural Orthostatic Tachycardia Syndrome (POTS). The main symptom of postural orthostatic hypotension (POTS) is a rapid and severe rise in heart rate (tachycardia) that happens shortly after standing up.

In particular, orthostatic tachycardia occurs when, in the absence of other causes (such as acute dehydration, prolonged bed rest, or medication side effects), the heart rate increases within 10 minutes of standing up by 30 bpm or more in adults (or 40 bpm or more in adolescents).

Lightheadedness, dizziness, fainting or near-fainting, blurred vision, palpitations, exhaustion, exercise intolerance, headaches, and tachycardia upon standing are among symptoms commonly experienced by individuals with POTS.

These symptoms can last a long time and have a major effect on how you live your life and how good you feel overall. POTS can manifest on its own or as a comorbidity with other diseases or health issues, including diabetes, autoimmune disorders, neurological disorders, Ehlers-Danlos syndrome, or a host of others.

Although the precise reason behind POTS remains a mystery, it is believed to be associated with issues within the autonomic nerve system, which regulates involuntary biological processes including digestion, heart rate, and blood pressure. Improving quality of life and reducing symptoms are the goals of treatment for POTS.

Drugs to treat underlying causes of POTS or to increase blood volume may be part of the treatment plan, along with behavioral changes (such as consuming more fluids and salt), physical therapy, and symptom-controlling drugs (such as beta-blockers or vasoconstrictors).

CHAPTER ONE
Types Of POTS

Postural Orthostatic Tachycardia Syndrome (POTS) can be classified into different types based on various underlying mechanisms or associated conditions. Here are some recognized types of POTS:

• **Neuropathic POTS:** This type of POTS is associated with a neuropathic dysfunction, where there is impaired peripheral sympathetic nerve function. This dysfunction leads to inadequate vasoconstriction upon standing, causing blood pooling in the lower extremities and subsequent tachycardia as the body tries to compensate.

- **Hyperadrenergic POTS:** In this type, there is excessive sympathetic nervous system activity, resulting in elevated levels of norepinephrine (a stress hormone). People with hyperadrenergic POTS often experience more severe symptoms such as palpitations, anxiety, and hypertension in addition to the typical POTS symptoms.

- **Secondary POTS:** This refers to cases where POTS develops secondary to another medical condition, such as Ehlers-Danlos syndrome, diabetes mellitus, amyloidosis, sarcoidosis, or autoimmune diseases like Sjögren's syndrome and lupus. Secondary POTS may have different underlying mechanisms depending on the primary condition.

- **Joint Hypermobility Syndrome (JHS)-related POTS:** This subtype is associated with joint hypermobility and often overlaps with Ehlers-Danlos syndrome (EDS). The hypermobility of joints may contribute to the dysfunction of the autonomic nervous system seen in POTS.

- **Mast Cell Activation Syndrome (MCAS)-related POTS:** Some individuals with POTS may also have mast cell activation syndrome, where mast cells release excessive amounts of chemical mediators, leading to symptoms such as flushing, itching, and gastrointestinal disturbances, which can exacerbate POTS symptoms.

- **Autoimmune POTS:** In rare cases, POTS may be associated with autoimmune mechanisms, where the immune system mistakenly attacks components of the autonomic nervous system or receptors involved in regulating blood pressure and heart rate.

These types of POTS can overlap, and individuals may have characteristics of more than one subtype. The classification helps guide treatment approaches and understanding of the underlying pathophysiology in each case, although the exact cause of POTS can vary widely among individuals.

Symptoms And Diagnosis

Symptoms of POTS:

The symptoms of Postural Orthostatic Tachycardia Syndrome (POTS) can vary from person to person but typically include:

• **Orthostatic Intolerance:** Symptoms that worsen when standing upright and improve when lying down. These may include lightheadedness, dizziness, feeling faint, or actual fainting (syncope).

• **Tachycardia:** A heart rate increase of at least 30 beats per minute (or to over 120 bpm) within 10 minutes of standing up, without a corresponding drop in blood pressure.

• **Fatigue:** Persistent tiredness that is not relieved by rest.

• **Exercise Intolerance:** Difficulty exercising or feeling worse after physical exertion.

- **Palpitations:** Awareness of the heart beating, irregular heart rhythms, or a pounding sensation in the chest.

- **Headaches:** Often described as migraine-like or tension headaches.

- **Cognitive Difficulties:** Brain fog, difficulty concentrating, and memory problems.

- **Gastrointestinal Symptoms:** Nausea, abdominal pain, and other digestive issues.

- **Sleep Disturbances:** Insomnia or disrupted sleep patterns.

- **Temperature Dysregulation:** Cold extremities or intolerance to heat.

- **Blurred Vision:** Vision disturbances, especially upon standing.

- **Shortness of Breath:** Difficulty breathing, especially during or after physical activity.

Diagnosis of POTS:

Diagnosing POTS involves a thorough evaluation by a healthcare professional, typically a cardiologist or autonomic specialist. The diagnostic process may include:

- **Medical History:** A detailed history of symptoms, their onset, triggers, and any relevant medical conditions or family history.

- **Physical Examination:** This includes measuring heart rate and blood pressure in different positions (lying down, sitting, and standing) to assess for orthostatic changes.

- **Tilt Table Test (TTT):** A specialized test where the patient is strapped to a table and tilted to an upright position while heart rate and blood pressure are monitored. This helps to confirm the presence of orthostatic intolerance and tachycardia.

- **Autonomic Function Testing:** This may include other tests to assess autonomic nervous system function, such as QSART (quantitative sudomotor axon reflex test), Valsalva maneuver, and other specialized assessments.

- **Blood Tests:** These may be done to rule out other conditions that can mimic POTS or contribute to its symptoms, such as thyroid disorders, autoimmune diseases, or electrolyte imbalances.

- **Cardiac Evaluation:** Echocardiogram and/or cardiac stress testing may be performed to evaluate heart function and rule out structural heart disease.

- **Monitoring Symptoms:** Sometimes, a symptom diary or continuous heart rate monitoring over several hours or days may be used to capture fluctuations in symptoms.

Once diagnosed, treatment is tailored to manage symptoms and improve quality of life, which may involve lifestyle modifications, medications, physical therapy, and occasionally other interventions depending on the underlying cause and severity of symptoms.

CHAPTER TWO
Causes And Risk Factors

Postural Orthostatic Tachycardia Syndrome (POTS) is a complex disorder with various factors contributing to its development. While the exact cause of POTS is not always clear, several potential causes and risk factors have been identified:

1. Autonomic Nervous System Dysfunction: POTS is often associated with dysfunction of the autonomic nervous system (ANS), which regulates involuntary bodily functions such as heart rate, blood pressure, digestion, and temperature control. In POTS, there is typically impaired regulation of blood flow and heart rate when moving from a lying down to a standing position, leading to symptoms of orthostatic intolerance.

2. Volume Dysregulation: Some individuals with POTS may have problems with blood volume regulation. This can include inadequate blood volume, excessive pooling of blood in the lower extremities upon standing, or abnormal vascular responsiveness.

3. Endocrine Abnormalities: Hormonal imbalances, such as low levels of aldosterone or abnormalities in norepinephrine and epinephrine levels, have been implicated in some cases of POTS.

4. Immune System Dysfunction: There is evidence suggesting that autoimmune mechanisms may play a role in some individuals with POTS. Autoimmune diseases like Sjögren's syndrome, lupus, or autoimmune autonomic ganglionopathy can cause or contribute to POTS symptoms.

5. Genetic Factors: There may be a genetic predisposition to developing POTS, as it can occur in families. Variants in genes involved in autonomic function or connective tissue disorders (such as Ehlers-Danlos syndrome) have been associated with POTS in some cases.

6. Joint Hypermobility: POTS is often seen in individuals with joint hypermobility syndromes like Ehlers-Danlos syndrome (EDS). Connective tissue abnormalities in these syndromes may affect blood vessel and autonomic nerve function, contributing to POTS symptoms.

7. Viral Infections: Some cases of POTS appear to be triggered by viral illnesses, such as Epstein-Barr virus (EBV), which can lead to an autoimmune response or affect the autonomic nervous system.

8. Postural Deconditioning: Prolonged bed rest or physical deconditioning can lead to orthostatic intolerance and potentially contribute to the development or exacerbation of POTS symptoms.

Risk Factors:

• **Age and Gender:** POTS predominantly affects younger individuals, often women of childbearing age, though it can occur in men and children as well.

• **Hormonal Changes:** POTS symptoms may worsen during menstrual periods, pregnancy, or with hormonal changes associated with puberty or menopause.

• **Prior Trauma or Surgery:** In some cases, trauma, surgery, or significant illness can trigger the onset of POTS symptoms.

• **Psychological Factors:** Stress and anxiety can exacerbate symptoms in some individuals with POTS, though they are not considered a direct cause.

Understanding these potential causes and risk factors can help healthcare providers diagnose POTS more accurately and develop appropriate treatment plans tailored to individual needs.

Pathophysiology Of POTS

The pathophysiology of Postural Orthostatic Tachycardia Syndrome (POTS) involves complex interactions between various physiological systems, primarily focusing on dysfunctions within the autonomic nervous system (ANS) and cardiovascular regulatory mechanisms. Here are the key aspects of POTS pathophysiology:

Autonomic Nervous System Dysfunction:

• **Sympathetic Nervous System (SNS) and Parasympathetic Nervous System (PNS) Imbalance:** One of the central features of POTS is an imbalance in the autonomic nervous system, particularly involving the sympathetic and parasympathetic branches. Normally, the SNS increases heart rate and constricts blood vessels to maintain blood pressure when standing up, while the PNS works to oppose these effects and maintain balance. In POTS, there is often excessive sympathetic tone or inadequate compensatory responses from the autonomic nervous system upon assuming an upright posture.

Impaired Orthostatic Tolerance:

• **Inadequate Vasoconstriction:** Upon standing, individuals with POTS often exhibit inadequate vasoconstriction in the lower limbs, leading to pooling of blood and decreased venous return to the heart. This triggers a compensatory increase in heart rate (tachycardia) to maintain cardiac output and blood pressure.

• **Hypovolemia or Altered Blood Volume Regulation:** Some individuals with POTS may have abnormalities in blood volume regulation, such as reduced blood volume or altered plasma volume, contributing to orthostatic intolerance.

Cardiovascular Responses:

- **Tachycardia:** The hallmark feature of POTS is a rapid increase in heart rate upon standing (orthostatic tachycardia), which can be excessive (typically an increase of 30 beats per minute or more).

- **Reduced Cardiac Output:** Despite the tachycardic response, some individuals with POTS may have reduced cardiac output or inefficient heart function, particularly during orthostatic stress.

Neurohormonal Dysregulation:

- **Norepinephrine and Epinephrine:** Dysregulation in the release and clearance of norepinephrine (NE) and epinephrine (EPI), catecholamines that play a crucial role in regulating heart rate and blood pressure, is common in POTS. Some individuals may have elevated levels of circulating catecholamines, contributing to symptoms of palpitations, anxiety, and hypertension.

• **Renin-Angiotensin-Aldosterone System (RAAS):** Alterations in the RAAS, which regulates blood pressure and fluid balance, may also contribute to the pathophysiology of POTS, particularly in cases associated with hypovolemia or blood volume dysregulation.

Hormonal and Immunological Factors:

• **Hormonal Fluctuations:** POTS symptoms may worsen during hormonal changes, such as menstrual cycles, pregnancy, or with changes in estrogen and progesterone levels.

• **Autoimmune Mechanisms:** In some individuals, POTS may be associated with autoimmune disorders or immune-mediated dysfunctions affecting the autonomic nervous system.

Genetic and Environmental Factors:

- **Genetic Predisposition:** There may be a genetic component to POTS, with certain genetic variants potentially predisposing individuals to autonomic dysfunction or connective tissue disorders (like Ehlers-Danlos syndrome) that are often associated with POTS.

- **Environmental Triggers:** Viral infections, physical trauma, surgery, or prolonged bed rest may trigger or exacerbate symptoms of POTS in susceptible individuals.

Understanding the multifaceted nature of POTS pathophysiology is crucial for developing effective treatment strategies aimed at improving symptoms and quality of life for individuals affected by this challenging syndrome. Treatment approaches often involve a combination of lifestyle modifications, medications to manage symptoms, and targeted therapies addressing underlying autonomic and cardiovascular dysfunctions.

CHAPTER THREE
How Diet Affects POTS Symptoms & Nutritional Needs Of POTS Patients

Diet can significantly impact the symptoms and overall well-being of individuals with Postural Orthostatic Tachycardia Syndrome (POTS). Managing dietary intake can help mitigate symptoms and improve quality of life. Here's how diet affects POTS symptoms and the nutritional needs of POTS patients:

Impact of Diet on POTS Symptoms:

Fluid and Electrolyte Balance:

• **Hydration:** Adequate fluid intake is crucial to maintain blood volume and prevent dehydration, which can worsen symptoms of orthostatic intolerance. POTS patients often benefit from increased fluid intake, including water, electrolyte-rich fluids (like sports drinks with sodium), and sometimes intravenous fluids under medical supervision.

- **Salt Intake:** Increasing dietary salt (sodium) can help expand blood volume and improve orthostatic symptoms. POTS patients are often advised to consume higher amounts of salt than the general population, under guidance from a healthcare provider, to counteract the tendency for blood pooling and orthostatic intolerance.

Meal Composition and Timing:

- **Balanced Meals:** Eating regular, balanced meals can help stabilize blood sugar levels and prevent postprandial hypotension (low blood pressure after eating), which can exacerbate POTS symptoms. Meals should include complex carbohydrates, lean proteins, and healthy fats.

- **Avoiding Large Meals:** Large meals can trigger symptoms in some POTS patients due to increased blood flow to the digestive system. Eating smaller, more frequent meals throughout the day may be beneficial.

Caffeine and Stimulants:

- **Caffeine Intake:** Caffeine can exacerbate tachycardia and anxiety symptoms in some individuals with POTS. It may be advisable to limit or avoid caffeine-containing beverages like coffee, tea, and certain sodas.

Alcohol and Dehydration:

- **Alcohol:** Alcohol can cause dehydration and worsen symptoms such as dizziness and fatigue. POTS patients are typically advised to consume alcohol in moderation or avoid it altogether.

Nutrient Deficiencies:

- **Micronutrients:** POTS patients may be at risk for deficiencies in certain vitamins and minerals, such as vitamin B12, folate, iron, and magnesium. A balanced diet rich in fruits, vegetables, whole grains, and lean proteins can help address these nutritional needs.

Nutritional Needs of POTS Patients:

Salt and Fluids:

- Ensuring adequate hydration with electrolyte-rich fluids.

- Consuming sufficient dietary salt to maintain blood volume and blood pressure stability.

Balanced Diet:

- Emphasizing whole foods, including fruits, vegetables, whole grains, lean proteins (like poultry, fish, beans), and healthy fats (like olive oil, avocados).

- Avoiding processed foods high in sugar, unhealthy fats, and artificial additives.

Supplements:

- In some cases, supplements may be recommended to address specific deficiencies identified through blood tests. This might include iron, vitamin D, or magnesium supplements, among others.

Meal Timing and Frequency:

- Eating smaller, more frequent meals to prevent large fluctuations in blood pressure and heart rate.

- Avoiding prolonged fasting, which can exacerbate symptoms.

Individualized Approach:

- Nutritional needs can vary among individuals with POTS, so it's important for patients to work closely with healthcare providers, such as dietitians or specialists familiar with POTS, to develop a personalized nutrition plan.

A well-balanced diet that supports hydration, electrolyte balance, and stable blood sugar levels can help manage symptoms and improve overall health in individuals with POTS. Adjustments to diet and lifestyle should be made in consultation with healthcare professionals to ensure they align with individual needs and goals.

Creating A POTS-Friendly Meal Plan

Creating a POTS-friendly meal plan involves focusing on foods and beverages that support hydration, stabilize blood sugar levels, and provide essential nutrients without exacerbating symptoms like tachycardia or digestive discomfort. Here's a sample meal plan tailored for someone with Postural Orthostatic Tachycardia Syndrome (POTS):

Breakfast:

Option 1:

- Greek yogurt with sliced bananas, a sprinkle of nuts or seeds (like almonds or chia seeds), and a drizzle of honey.

- Herbal tea or decaffeinated coffee.

Option 2:

- Oatmeal made with water or almond milk, topped with berries (like strawberries or blueberries), a dollop of nut butter (like almond or peanut butter), and a dash of cinnamon.

- Coconut water or electrolyte-rich fruit juice (unsweetened).

Mid-Morning Snack:

Option 1:

- Apple slices with a small handful of nuts (like walnuts or cashews).

- Water with a pinch of salt.

Option 2:

- Rice cakes with hummus or avocado spread.

- Herbal tea or electrolyte drink.

Lunch:

Option 1:

- Grilled chicken or tofu salad with mixed greens, cherry tomatoes, cucumber slices, and a light vinaigrette dressing (olive oil and vinegar).

- Quinoa or brown rice on the side.

- Water or coconut water.

Option 2:

- Whole grain wrap with turkey or roast beef, lettuce, tomato, avocado, and a spread of hummus or mustard.

- Carrot and celery sticks with hummus for dipping.

- Herbal tea or electrolyte drink.

Afternoon Snack:

Option 1:

- Smoothie made with spinach, berries (like raspberries or blackberries), banana, almond milk, and a scoop of protein powder or Greek yogurt.

- Water with electrolyte mix.

Option 2:

- Cottage cheese with sliced peaches or pineapple.

- Herbal tea or electrolyte-rich beverage.

Dinner:

Option 1:

- Baked salmon with steamed asparagus and quinoa.

- Mixed green salad with a light vinaigrette.

- Water or coconut water.

Option 2:

- Stir-fried tofu or shrimp with mixed vegetables (bell peppers, broccoli, snap peas) and brown rice.

- Water with a pinch of salt.

Evening Snack:

Option 1:

- Plain popcorn sprinkled with nutritional yeast or a dash of sea salt.

- Herbal tea or decaffeinated beverage.

Option 2:

- Sliced pear with a small piece of cheese (like cheddar or goat cheese).

- Water or herbal tea.

General Tips:

- **Hydration:** Drink plenty of fluids throughout the day, including water, electrolyte-rich beverages, and herbal teas.

- **Salt Intake:** Add a pinch of salt to meals or consume salted snacks to maintain electrolyte balance.

- **Frequent Meals:** Aim for smaller, more frequent meals and snacks to prevent large fluctuations in blood pressure and heart rate.

- **Avoid Triggers:** Limit or avoid caffeine, alcohol, and heavily processed foods that can exacerbate symptoms.

This meal plan provides a balanced mix of carbohydrates, proteins, healthy fats, vitamins, and minerals to support overall health and manage POTS symptoms effectively.

CHAPTER FOUR
Grocery Shopping Tips

When shopping for groceries with POTS in mind, it's important to focus on items that support hydration, stabilize blood sugar levels, and provide essential nutrients without exacerbating symptoms. Here are some grocery shopping tips tailored for individuals with Postural Orthostatic Tachycardia Syndrome (POTS):

1. Hydration and Electrolytes:

- **Electrolyte-rich beverages:** Look for electrolyte drinks, coconut water, or electrolyte powders that can help maintain hydration and electrolyte balance.

- **Fruits:** Choose hydrating fruits like watermelon, oranges, grapes, and berries.

- **Vegetables:** Opt for hydrating vegetables such as cucumbers, celery, lettuce, and bell peppers.

2. Dietary Staples:

- **Whole Grains:** Include whole grains like quinoa, brown rice, oats, and whole grain breads for sustained energy and fiber.

- **Lean Proteins:** Select lean proteins such as chicken breast, turkey, tofu, fish, and beans to support muscle function and energy levels.

- **Healthy Fats:** Choose sources of healthy fats such as avocados, nuts (like almonds and walnuts), seeds (like chia and flaxseed), and olive oil.

3. Snack Options:

- **Nuts and Seeds:** Stock up on almonds, cashews, walnuts, chia seeds, and pumpkin seeds for quick, nutrient-dense snacks.

- **Dried Fruits:** Look for unsweetened dried fruits like raisins, apricots, and cranberries for natural sweetness and energy.

- **Whole Grain Crackers:** Consider whole grain crackers or rice cakes as a base for snacks with toppings like nut butter, hummus, or cheese.

4. Beverages:

• **Herbal Teas:** Choose caffeine-free herbal teas for hydration and relaxation.

• **Decaffeinated Options:** Opt for decaffeinated coffee and tea if you enjoy these beverages but need to minimize caffeine intake.

• **Low-Sugar Drinks:** Select unsweetened almond milk, coconut water, or sparkling water as alternatives to sugary drinks.

5. Fresh Produce:

• **Leafy Greens:** Include spinach, kale, and Swiss chard for vitamins, minerals, and antioxidants.

• **Colorful Vegetables:** Pick up a variety of colorful vegetables such as carrots, bell peppers, broccoli, and tomatoes for diverse nutrients.

- **Seasonal Fruits:** Choose seasonal fruits like apples, pears, citrus fruits, and berries for freshness and flavor.

6. Other Considerations:

- **Salt and Seasonings:** Ensure you have iodized salt or sea salt for adding to meals as needed to support blood pressure stability.

- **Canned Goods:** Consider canned beans (low-sodium varieties if available), canned tuna or salmon, and canned tomatoes for quick meal options.

- **Frozen Foods:** Have frozen fruits and vegetables on hand for convenience and to retain nutrients. Frozen berries are great for smoothies.

Tips for Shopping:

- **Plan Ahead:** Make a list based on your meal plan and ensure you have everything you need to avoid extra trips.

- **Read Labels:** Check labels for added sugars, sodium content, and artificial ingredients, especially in packaged and processed foods.

By focusing on nutrient-dense foods, hydration, and balanced meals, you can help manage POTS symptoms and support overall health through your grocery choices. Adjust your shopping habits based on personal preferences and specific dietary recommendations from healthcare providers.

Meal Prep And Cooking Tips

Meal prep and cooking can be challenging for individuals with POTS due to symptoms like fatigue, dizziness, and difficulty standing for long periods. Here are some meal prep and cooking tips tailored for managing POTS:

Meal Prep Tips:

Plan Ahead:

• **Weekly Menu:** Plan your meals for the week, including breakfast, lunch, dinner, and snacks. This helps you organize your shopping list and streamline meal prep.

• **Batch Cooking:** Cook larger portions of meals that can be divided into individual servings and stored for quick reheating throughout the week.

Simplify Recipes:

• **One-Pot Meals:** Choose recipes that require minimal preparation and cooking time, such as soups, stews, and casseroles.

• **Sheet Pan Meals:** Prepare meals using a sheet pan, roasting vegetables and protein together for easy cleanup and fewer dishes.

Prep Ingredients:

- **Chop Veggies:** Wash and chop vegetables in advance, storing them in containers or resealable bags for easy access during meal prep.

- **Pre-Cook Proteins:** Cook proteins like chicken breast, tofu, or ground turkey ahead of time, then portion and refrigerate or freeze for quick meals.

Use Convenience Foods:

- **Frozen Vegetables:** Opt for frozen vegetables, which are already washed and chopped, saving time and effort during meal prep.

- **Canned Beans and Tomatoes:** Stock up on canned beans (rinsed to reduce sodium) and diced tomatoes for quick additions to soups, stews, and salads.

Cooking Tips:

Cooking Methods:

• **Slow Cooker:** Utilize a slow cooker for hands-off cooking. Prepare ingredients in the morning and come home to a ready-made meal.

• **Instant Pot:** Pressure cookers like the Instant Pot can quickly cook meals like soups, grains, and proteins, reducing overall cooking time.

Avoid Standing:

• **Use Stools or Chairs:** Place a stool or chair in the kitchen to sit while chopping vegetables or stirring pots to minimize fatigue and dizziness.

• **Sit When Possible:** When cooking, use kitchen appliances at countertop height to minimize the need for bending or standing.

Hydration and Snacks:

- **Stay Hydrated:** Keep a bottle of water or electrolyte drink nearby to sip on while cooking to maintain hydration levels.

- **Prepared Snacks:** Have ready-to-eat snacks available, like nuts, dried fruits, or cut-up vegetables, to keep energy levels stable while cooking.

Break Tasks into Smaller Steps:

- **Pace Yourself:** Divide meal prep and cooking tasks into smaller segments. Take breaks as needed to avoid overexertion and manage symptoms.

Meal Assembly:

- **Assembly Style:** Prepare components of meals separately (e.g., grains, proteins, vegetables) and assemble them into complete meals when ready to eat or pack for work or outings.

- **Portion Control:** Use portion-sized containers for storing meals, making it easier to grab and go without additional preparation.

General Tips:

- **Listen to Your Body:** Pay attention to your symptoms and adjust your meal prep and cooking routine accordingly. Rest as needed to prevent exacerbation of symptoms.

- **Enlist Help:** Involve family members or friends in meal prep and cooking tasks when possible to share the workload and make the process more manageable.

- **Adapt Recipes:** Modify recipes to suit your dietary preferences and restrictions, ensuring meals are enjoyable and nutritious.

By incorporating these meal prep and cooking tips, individuals with POTS can simplify their meal planning, reduce physical strain, and maintain a balanced diet to support overall health and manage symptoms effectively. Adjust strategies based on personal needs and consult healthcare providers for tailored dietary advice.

CHAPTER FIVE
Food Sensitivities And Allergies

Food sensitivities and allergies can significantly impact individuals with Postural Orthostatic Tachycardia Syndrome (POTS), as they can exacerbate symptoms or trigger immune responses that worsen overall health. Here are considerations and tips for managing food sensitivities and allergies in relation to POTS:

1. Identifying Food Sensitivities and Allergies:

- **Common Triggers:** Keep track of foods that seem to worsen POTS symptoms or cause allergic reactions. Common triggers include gluten, dairy, soy, eggs, nuts, and shellfish.

- **Symptom Journal:** Maintain a food and symptom journal to identify patterns and potential triggers. Note any symptoms like gastrointestinal discomfort, headaches, fatigue, or worsening of orthostatic symptoms after consuming specific foods.

- **Consultation:** Work with a healthcare provider, such as an allergist or dietitian, to conduct allergy testing or elimination diets to pinpoint specific food sensitivities or allergies.

2. Managing Food Sensitivities and Allergies:

• **Avoidance:** Once identified, strictly avoid foods that trigger allergic reactions or worsen POTS symptoms.

• **Reading Labels:** Carefully read food labels to identify potential allergens or ingredients that may cause sensitivities.

• **Cross-Contamination:** Be cautious of cross-contamination in kitchens or restaurants, especially if you have severe allergies. Communicate dietary needs clearly when dining out.

• **Alternative Ingredients:** Substitute allergenic ingredients with alternatives. For example, use non-dairy milk alternatives (like almond milk or oat milk) instead of cow's milk.

- **Meal Preparation:** Prepare meals at home to have better control over ingredients and minimize exposure to allergens.

3. Nutritional Considerations:

- **Nutrient Replacement:** If eliminating certain foods affects nutrient intake, work with a dietitian to ensure adequate replacement with alternative sources.

- **Balanced Diet:** Maintain a balanced diet by focusing on whole, unprocessed foods that do not trigger allergies or sensitivities. Emphasize fruits, vegetables, lean proteins, and gluten-free grains as appropriate.

- **Supplements:** Consider supplements if dietary restrictions impact nutrient absorption or intake, such as calcium and vitamin D for dairy-free diets.

4. Meal Planning and Cooking:

- **Allergy-Friendly Recipes:** Explore allergy-friendly cookbooks or websites for recipes that cater to specific dietary restrictions.

- **Meal Prep:** Use meal prep techniques to ensure allergen-free meals are readily available, minimizing the risk of accidental exposure.

- **Storage:** Store allergen-free ingredients separately and clearly label containers to avoid confusion.

5. Educating Others:

- **Family and Friends:** Educate those around you, including family members, friends, and caregivers, about your food allergies and sensitivities to prevent accidental exposure.

- **School or Work:** Communicate dietary needs with school or workplace personnel to ensure accommodations are made when necessary.

General Tips:

• **Emergency Plan:** Have an emergency action plan in place for severe allergic reactions (anaphylaxis), including carrying prescribed medications (like epinephrine auto-injectors) if needed.

• **Medical Alert:** Wear a medical alert bracelet or necklace specifying food allergies or medical conditions related to POTS.

• **Regular Monitoring:** Regularly review and update your allergy management plan with healthcare providers as needed.

By proactively managing food sensitivities and allergies, individuals with POTS can reduce symptom flare-ups and maintain a healthy diet that supports overall well-being. Collaboration with healthcare professionals is essential to ensure dietary changes are safe and effective.

Gluten-Free And Dairy-Free Options

For individuals with Postural Orthostatic Tachycardia Syndrome (POTS) who also need to follow a gluten-free and dairy-free diet due to sensitivities or allergies, it's essential to focus on nutritious alternatives that support overall health and symptom management. Here are some gluten-free and dairy-free options and alternatives to consider:

Gluten-Free Options:

Grains and Starches:

- **Quinoa:** A versatile grain high in protein and fiber.

- **Brown Rice:** Nutritious and easy to digest.

- **Buckwheat:** Despite its name, buckwheat is gluten-free and can be used in porridge, pancakes, or as a substitute for rice.

Gluten-Free Flours:

- **Almond Flour:** Ground almonds that add richness to baked goods.

- **Coconut Flour:** High in fiber and adds a slight sweetness to recipes.

- **Oat Flour (if certified gluten-free):** Ground oats suitable for baking and cooking.

Breads and Wraps:

- **Gluten-Free Bread:** Look for varieties made from rice, quinoa, or almond flour.

- **Lettuce Wraps:** Use large lettuce leaves as a wrap alternative for sandwiches and wraps.

Pasta and Noodles:

- **Brown Rice Pasta:** Cooks similarly to wheat pasta and available in various shapes.

- **Zucchini Noodles (Zoodles):** Spiralized zucchini strands as a low-carb alternative.

Snacks:

- **Rice Cakes:** Plain or flavored rice cakes are a gluten-free snack option.

- **Popcorn:** Plain popcorn kernels are naturally gluten-free.

Dairy-Free Options:

Milk Alternatives:

- **Almond Milk:** Mild, nutty flavor suitable for drinking and cooking.

- **Coconut Milk:** Rich and creamy, ideal for curries and desserts.

- **Oat Milk:** Creamy texture with a neutral taste, great for coffee and baking.

Cheese Alternatives:

- **Nutritional Yeast:** Provides a cheesy flavor and is rich in B vitamins.

- **Dairy-Free Cheese:** Options made from nuts (like cashew or almond) or soy, available in slices or shredded forms.

Yogurt Alternatives:

- **Coconut Yogurt:** Made from coconut milk, available in plain or flavored varieties.

- **Almond Milk Yogurt:** Dairy-free alternative with a creamy texture.

Butter Alternatives:

- **Coconut Oil:** Substitute for butter in cooking and baking.

- **Avocado:** Mashed avocado can replace butter on toast or as a spread.

Ice Cream Alternatives:

- **Sorbet:** Fruit-based frozen dessert with a refreshing taste.

- **Coconut Milk Ice Cream:** Creamy texture similar to traditional ice cream.

Meal and Snack Ideas:

- **Breakfast:** Quinoa porridge with almond milk and berries, or gluten-free oats with coconut yogurt and nuts.

- **Lunch:** Brown rice pasta salad with mixed vegetables and olive oil dressing, or lettuce wraps with turkey, avocado, and tomato.

- **Dinner:** Grilled salmon with quinoa and steamed broccoli, or stir-fried tofu with rice noodles and vegetables in a gluten-free soy sauce.

- **Snacks:** Fresh fruit with nut butter, rice cakes with dairy-free cheese, or popcorn seasoned with herbs and nutritional yeast.

By choosing gluten-free and dairy-free options wisely, individuals with POTS can enjoy a varied and nutritious diet while managing their symptoms effectively. It's important to work with a healthcare provider or dietitian to ensure dietary needs are met and nutritional balance is maintained.

CHAPTER SIX
Vegetarian And Vegan Diets

Following a vegetarian or vegan diet can be beneficial for individuals with Postural Orthostatic Tachycardia Syndrome (POTS), as these diets can be rich in plant-based nutrients while avoiding potential triggers like dairy or excessive animal fats. Here's a guide to vegetarian and vegan options tailored for managing POTS:

Vegetarian Options:

Plant-Based Proteins:

• **Legumes:** Beans (like chickpeas, black beans, and kidney beans), lentils, and peas are rich sources of protein, fiber, and essential nutrients.

• **Tofu and Tempeh:** Soy-based products that provide versatile protein options for stir-fries, salads, and sandwiches.

- **Eggs:** If included, eggs provide complete protein and essential vitamins. Consider free-range or organic options.

Whole Grains:

- **Quinoa:** High in protein and fiber, quinoa is a nutritious base for salads, bowls, and side dishes.

- **Brown Rice, Whole Wheat Pasta, and Oats:** These provide complex carbohydrates for sustained energy without gluten.

Dairy Alternatives:

• **Plant-Based Milks:** Choose almond milk, soy milk, oat milk, or rice milk as alternatives to cow's milk.

• **Cheese Alternatives:** Look for vegetarian cheeses made from nuts (like cashews) or soy, available in various flavors and textures.

Fruits and Vegetables:

• **Leafy Greens:** Spinach, kale, and Swiss chard are rich in vitamins and minerals.

• **Colorful Vegetables:** Bell peppers, carrots, tomatoes, and broccoli provide antioxidants and essential nutrients.

Healthy Fats:

• **Nuts and Seeds:** Almonds, walnuts, chia seeds, and flaxseeds are excellent sources of omega-3 fatty acids and protein.

• **Avocado and Olive Oil:** Incorporate these heart-healthy fats into salads, spreads, and cooking.

Vegan Options:

Protein Sources:

• **Legumes and Beans:** Include a variety such as lentils, chickpeas, black beans, and edamame for protein and fiber.

• **Seitan and Soy Products:** Seitan (wheat gluten) and soy-based products like tempeh and tofu provide versatile protein options.

Grains and Starches:

- **Quinoa, Brown Rice, and Buckwheat:** These gluten-free options are nutrient-dense and suitable for a vegan diet.

- **Whole Wheat Pasta and Millet:** Incorporate these grains into meals for added variety and nutrition.

Plant-Based Milks and Dairy Alternatives:

- **Almond, Soy, Coconut, and Oat Milk:** These can be used in cooking, baking, or as beverages.

- **Vegan Cheeses:** Look for dairy-free cheeses made from nuts, soy, or coconut for sandwiches, pizzas, and snacks.

Fruits and Vegetables:

- **Fresh Produce:** Incorporate a variety of seasonal fruits and vegetables for vitamins, minerals, and antioxidants.

- **Dark Leafy Greens:** Spinach, kale, and collard greens are excellent sources of iron and calcium.

Healthy Fats:

- **Nuts, Seeds, and Avocado:** These provide essential fatty acids and can be added to salads, smoothies, or eaten as snacks.

- **Coconut Oil and Olive Oil:** Use these plant-based oils for cooking and dressing salads.

Meal and Snack Ideas:

- **Breakfast:** Smoothie bowls with plant-based protein powder, chia seeds, and mixed berries, or avocado toast on gluten-free bread with tomato and nutritional yeast.

- **Lunch:** Quinoa salad with mixed greens, chickpeas, cucumber, and tahini dressing, or tofu stir-fry with vegetables and brown rice.

- **Dinner:** Lentil soup with whole grain bread, or stuffed bell peppers with quinoa, black beans, and vegan cheese.

- **Snacks:** Hummus with carrot sticks, trail mix with nuts and dried fruit, or sliced apple with almond butter.

Tips for Balanced Nutrition:

• **Protein Balance:** Ensure each meal includes a source of protein (legumes, tofu, tempeh, etc.) to support muscle function and energy levels.

• **Iron and B12:** Monitor intake of iron-rich foods (like beans and leafy greens) and consider supplementation or fortified foods for vitamin B12, which may be lacking in vegan diets.

• **Omega-3s:** Incorporate flaxseeds, chia seeds, walnuts, or algae-based supplements to meet omega-3 fatty acid needs.

By incorporating a variety of nutrient-dense foods and planning meals thoughtfully, individuals with POTS can maintain a healthy vegetarian or vegan diet that supports overall well-being and helps manage symptoms effectively. Consulting with a healthcare provider or dietitian can provide personalized guidance based on individual needs and health goals.

Energizing Smoothies Recipes For Breakfast

Energizing smoothies can be an excellent addition to the diet of individuals with Postural Orthostatic Tachycardia Syndrome (POTS), providing essential nutrients, hydration, and energy without exacerbating symptoms. Here are three energizing smoothie recipes tailored for managing POTS:

1. Green Power Smoothie:

Ingredients:

- 1 cup spinach or kale (fresh or frozen)
- 1/2 cup cucumber, peeled and chopped
- 1/2 cup pineapple chunks (fresh or frozen)
- 1/2 banana (fresh or frozen)
- 1 tablespoon chia seeds
- 1 cup coconut water or almond milk (unsweetened)
- Ice cubes (optional)

Instructions:

- Place spinach or kale, cucumber, pineapple, banana, and chia seeds into a blender.
- Add coconut water or almond milk.
- Blend until smooth and creamy.
- Add ice cubes if desired and blend again until well combined.
- Pour into a glass and enjoy immediately.
- **Benefits:** This smoothie is packed with hydrating coconut water, leafy greens for vitamins and minerals, and pineapple and banana for natural sweetness and energy. Chia seeds add fiber and omega-3 fatty acids for sustained energy.

2. Berry Blast Smoothie:

Ingredients:

- 1/2 cup mixed berries (such as strawberries, blueberries, raspberries)
- 1/2 cup plain Greek yogurt or dairy-free yogurt alternative
- 1/2 banana (fresh or frozen)
- 1 tablespoon almond butter or peanut butter
- 1 tablespoon honey or maple syrup (optional, for sweetness)
- 1 cup almond milk or coconut water
- Ice cubes (optional)

Instructions:

- Combine mixed berries, yogurt, banana, almond butter, and honey or maple syrup in a blender.
- Add almond milk or coconut water.
- Blend until smooth and creamy.
- Add ice cubes if desired and blend again until well combined.

- Pour into a glass and serve immediately.
- **Benefits:** This smoothie provides antioxidants from berries, protein from Greek yogurt or dairy-free alternative, and healthy fats and additional protein from almond butter or peanut butter. It's a balanced option for sustained energy.

3. Tropical Sunshine Smoothie

Ingredients:

- 1/2 cup mango chunks (fresh or frozen)
- 1/2 cup pineapple chunks (fresh or frozen)
- 1/2 banana (fresh or frozen)
- Juice of 1/2 lime
- 1 tablespoon flaxseed meal or hemp seeds

- 1 cup coconut water or orange juice (unsweetened)
- Ice cubes (optional)

Instructions:

- Place mango, pineapple, banana, lime juice, and flaxseed meal or hemp seeds into a blender.
- Add coconut water or orange juice.
- Blend until smooth and creamy.
- Add ice cubes if desired and blend again until well combined.
- Pour into a glass and enjoy immediately.
- **Benefits:** This smoothie is refreshing and hydrating with tropical fruits and coconut water or orange juice. Flaxseed meal or hemp seeds add omega-3 fatty acids and fiber for sustained energy and satiety.

Tips for Customizing Smoothies:

- **Protein Boost:** Add a scoop of protein powder (such as pea protein or hemp protein) to any of these smoothies for an additional protein boost.

- **Hydration:** Adjust the consistency by adding more liquid (water, coconut water, or juice) for a thinner smoothie or less for a thicker texture.

- **Nutrient Variety:** Experiment with different fruits, vegetables, and seeds to vary flavors and nutritional benefits.

These energizing smoothies can be enjoyed as part of a balanced diet to support energy levels, hydration, and overall well-being for individuals managing POTS. Adjust ingredients based on personal preferences and dietary needs, and consult with a healthcare provider or dietitian for personalized advice.

High-Protein Breakfast Bowls Recipes

High-protein breakfast bowls are excellent for individuals with Postural Orthostatic Tachycardia Syndrome (POTS) as they provide sustained energy and essential nutrients. Here are three nutritious and delicious recipes for high-protein breakfast bowls:

1. Quinoa and Egg Breakfast Bowl:

Ingredients:

- 1/2 cup cooked quinoa
- 1 boiled egg, sliced
- 1/2 avocado, sliced
- Handful of cherry tomatoes, halved
- Handful of spinach or kale
- 1 tablespoon hummus or tahini
- Optional: Sprinkle of hemp seeds or pumpkin seeds
- Salt and pepper to taste

Instructions:

- Cook quinoa according to package instructions and allow to cool slightly.
- In a bowl, layer cooked quinoa, sliced boiled egg, avocado slices, cherry tomatoes, and spinach or kale.
- Drizzle with hummus or tahini.
- Sprinkle with hemp seeds or pumpkin seeds for added protein and texture.
- Season with salt and pepper to taste.
- Enjoy your nutritious and protein-packed breakfast bowl!

Benefits: This breakfast bowl is rich in protein from quinoa and eggs, healthy fats from avocado, and vitamins and minerals from vegetables. Hummus or tahini adds flavor and additional protein.

2. Greek Yogurt and Berry Breakfast Bowl:

Ingredients:

- 1 cup plain Greek yogurt or dairy-free yogurt alternative
- 1/2 cup mixed berries (such as strawberries, blueberries, raspberries)
- 1/4 cup granola (look for gluten-free options if needed)
- 1 tablespoon almond butter or peanut butter
- Optional: Drizzle of honey or maple syrup

Instructions:

- Spoon Greek yogurt or dairy-free alternative into a bowl.
- Top with mixed berries and granola.
- Drizzle almond butter or peanut butter over the top.
- Optionally, add a drizzle of honey or maple syrup for sweetness.
- Mix gently to combine ingredients.

- Enjoy your creamy and protein-rich breakfast bowl!

Benefits: This bowl provides protein from Greek yogurt, antioxidants from berries, and healthy fats and fiber from almond butter or peanut butter. Granola adds crunch and additional nutrients.

3. Tofu and Vegetable Breakfast Bowl

Ingredients:

- 1/2 cup firm tofu, cubed
- 1/2 cup cooked quinoa or brown rice
- 1 cup mixed vegetables (such as bell peppers, spinach, zucchini)
- 1 tablespoon olive oil
- 1/2 teaspoon garlic powder
- Salt and pepper to taste
- Optional toppings: Sliced avocado, nutritional yeast, salsa

Instructions:

- Heat olive oil in a skillet over medium heat. Add cubed tofu and cook until lightly browned on all sides.
- Add mixed vegetables to the skillet and sauté until tender.
- Season with garlic powder, salt, and pepper to taste.
- In a bowl, layer cooked quinoa or brown rice, sautéed tofu and vegetables.
- Top with optional toppings like sliced avocado, nutritional yeast, or salsa.
- Mix gently to combine flavors and textures.
- Enjoy your savory and protein-packed breakfast bowl!

Benefits: This bowl is high in plant-based protein from tofu, fiber from quinoa or brown rice, and vitamins and minerals from mixed vegetables. It's a satisfying and nutritious breakfast option.

Tips for Customization:

- **Add Seeds:** Sprinkle hemp seeds, chia seeds, or flaxseeds over any of these bowls for an extra boost of protein and omega-3 fatty acids.
- **Greens:** Incorporate fresh spinach, kale, or arugula for added nutrients and fiber.
- **Sauce or Dressing:** Experiment with different sauces or dressings such as balsamic glaze, lemon tahini dressing, or yogurt-based sauces for added flavor.

These high-protein breakfast bowls are versatile and can be customized based on personal preferences and dietary needs. They provide a balanced combination of protein, carbohydrates, healthy fats, and essential nutrients to support energy levels and overall well-being for individuals managing POTS.

Adjust ingredients as needed and consult with a healthcare provider or dietitian for personalized recommendations.

Salt-Rich Breakfast Ideas Recipes

For individuals with Postural Orthostatic Tachycardia Syndrome (POTS), adding extra salt to the diet can help manage symptoms such as low blood pressure and orthostatic intolerance. Here are some salt-rich breakfast ideas that are nutritious and can provide the sodium needed:

1. Avocado Toast with Smoked Salmon

Ingredients:

- 2 slices of whole grain bread (gluten-free if needed)
- 1 ripe avocado
- 4 oz smoked salmon
- Lemon juice
- Salt and pepper to taste

- Optional toppings: Fresh dill, capers

Instructions:

- Toast the whole grain bread slices until golden brown.
- Mash the ripe avocado and spread it evenly on the toasted bread slices.
- Squeeze a bit of lemon juice over the avocado.
- Season with salt and pepper to taste.
- Top each slice with smoked salmon.
- Garnish with fresh dill and capers if desired.
- Serve immediately.

Benefits: This breakfast is rich in healthy fats from avocado and omega-3 fatty acids from smoked salmon. It's also high in sodium, which can help maintain blood pressure levels for POTS management.

2. Greek Yogurt Parfait with Nuts and Seeds:

Ingredients:

- 1 cup plain Greek yogurt or dairy-free yogurt alternative
- 1 tablespoon honey or maple syrup (optional for sweetness)
- 1/4 cup mixed nuts (such as almonds, walnuts, or cashews)
- 1 tablespoon chia seeds or flaxseeds
- Fresh berries or dried fruit for topping
- Pinch of salt

Instructions:

- In a bowl or glass, layer Greek yogurt with honey or maple syrup if using.
- Sprinkle mixed nuts and seeds (chia seeds or flaxseeds) over the yogurt.
- Add a pinch of salt over the nuts and seeds.
- Top with fresh berries or dried fruit.
- Serve immediately.

Benefits: Greek yogurt provides protein and probiotics, while nuts and seeds add healthy fats, fiber, and additional protein. The pinch of salt enhances flavor and provides essential sodium.

3. Breakfast Burrito with Beans and Cheese:

Ingredients:

- 1 large gluten-free or whole grain tortilla
- 1/2 cup canned black beans, rinsed and drained
- 1/4 cup shredded cheese (cheddar, mozzarella, or dairy-free alternative)
- 1/4 cup salsa
- Fresh spinach or lettuce leaves
- Pinch of salt
- Optional toppings: Avocado slices, sour cream or yogurt

Instructions:

- Heat the tortilla in a skillet or microwave until warm and pliable.
- Layer black beans, shredded cheese, salsa, and fresh spinach or lettuce leaves on the tortilla.
- Sprinkle a pinch of salt over the filling.
- Fold the sides of the tortilla over the filling to form a burrito.
- Optionally, top with avocado slices, sour cream, or yogurt.
- Serve immediately.

Benefits: This breakfast option provides protein and fiber from black beans, calcium from cheese (or calcium-fortified dairy-free cheese), and essential sodium from salt. It's a hearty and savory breakfast that can be customized with additional toppings.

Tips for Adding Salt-Rich Foods:

- **Olives:** Include olives or tapenade as a side or topping for extra saltiness.
- **Cured Meats:** Add small amounts of cured meats like prosciutto or bacon as part of a balanced breakfast.
- **Sauces and Condiments:** Use salt-rich sauces such as soy sauce, Worcestershire sauce, or hot sauce to enhance flavor.

By incorporating these salt-rich breakfast ideas into your morning routine, individuals with POTS can help manage symptoms related to low blood pressure and orthostatic intolerance. Adjust ingredients based on personal preferences and consult with a healthcare provider or dietitian for personalized dietary recommendations.

CHAPTER SEVEN
Light And Nourishing Salads Recipes For Lunch

Light and nourishing salads can be ideal for individuals with Postural Orthostatic Tachycardia Syndrome (POTS) as they provide hydration, essential nutrients, and can be customized to include ingredients that support overall health and symptom management. Here are three recipes for refreshing salads that are both light and nourishing:

1. Quinoa and Chickpea Salad:

Ingredients:

- 1 cup cooked quinoa, cooled
- 1 can chickpeas, rinsed and drained
- 1 cucumber, diced
- 1 bell pepper (any color), diced
- 1/4 cup red onion, thinly sliced
- Handful of cherry tomatoes, halved

- Handful of fresh parsley, chopped
- Juice of 1 lemon
- 2 tablespoons extra virgin olive oil
- Salt and pepper to taste

Instructions:

- In a large bowl, combine cooked quinoa, chickpeas, cucumber, bell pepper, red onion, cherry tomatoes, and parsley.
- In a small bowl, whisk together lemon juice and olive oil.
- Drizzle the dressing over the salad and toss gently to combine.
- Season with salt and pepper to taste.
- Serve chilled or at room temperature.

Benefits: This salad is rich in protein from quinoa and chickpeas, fiber from vegetables, and vitamins from fresh herbs and lemon juice. It's light yet filling, perfect for a nutritious meal.

2. Spinach and Berry Salad with Balsamic Vinaigrette:

Ingredients:

- 4 cups fresh spinach leaves
- 1 cup mixed berries (such as strawberries, blueberries, raspberries)
- 1/4 cup sliced almonds or walnuts
- 1/4 cup crumbled feta cheese or dairy-free alternative
- Balsamic vinaigrette dressing:
- 3 tablespoons balsamic vinegar
- 2 tablespoons extra virgin olive oil
- 1 teaspoon honey or maple syrup (optional for sweetness)
- Salt and pepper to taste

Instructions:

- In a large bowl, combine fresh spinach leaves, mixed berries, sliced almonds or walnuts, and crumbled feta cheese.

- In a small bowl or jar, whisk together balsamic vinegar, olive oil, and honey or maple syrup if using.
- Drizzle the dressing over the salad and toss gently to coat.
- Season with salt and pepper to taste.
- Serve immediately.

Benefits: This salad is packed with antioxidants from berries, iron and vitamins from spinach, and healthy fats from nuts and olive oil. The balsamic vinaigrette adds a tangy flavor without being heavy.

3. Asian-Inspired Edamame and Cabbage Salad

Ingredients:

- 2 cups shredded cabbage (green or purple)
- 1 cup shelled edamame, cooked and cooled

- 1 carrot, julienned or grated
- 1/4 cup sliced green onions
- Handful of cilantro leaves, chopped
- Sesame ginger dressing:
- 3 tablespoons rice vinegar
- 2 tablespoons soy sauce or tamari (gluten-free option)
- 1 tablespoon sesame oil
- 1 tablespoon honey or maple syrup
- 1 teaspoon grated ginger
- Optional: Toasted sesame seeds for garnish
- Salt and pepper to taste

Instructions:

- In a large bowl, combine shredded cabbage, edamame, carrot, green onions, and cilantro.
- In a small bowl or jar, whisk together rice vinegar, soy sauce or tamari,

sesame oil, honey or maple syrup, and grated ginger to make the dressing.
- Drizzle the dressing over the salad and toss gently to combine.
- Season with salt and pepper to taste.
- Garnish with toasted sesame seeds if desired.
- Serve chilled or at room temperature.

Benefits: This salad is rich in plant-based protein from edamame, fiber from cabbage and carrots, and antioxidants from cilantro and sesame seeds. The sesame ginger dressing adds a flavorful Asian-inspired touch.

Tips for Customization:

• **Protein Boost:** Add grilled chicken, tofu, or quinoa to any of these salads for an extra protein boost.

- **Grains:** Incorporate cooked grains like brown rice or farro for added texture and nutrients.

- **Fruit Variations:** Experiment with seasonal fruits like apples, pears, or mangoes in salads for a sweet and savory combination.

These lights and nourishing salad recipes are versatile and can be adjusted based on personal preferences and dietary needs. They provide a variety of nutrients essential for managing POTS symptoms while offering refreshing flavors and textures. Adjust ingredients as needed and consult with a healthcare provider or dietitian for personalized dietary recommendations.

Protein-Packed Sandwiches And Wraps Recipes

Creating protein-packed sandwiches and wraps can be a great option for individuals with Postural Orthostatic Tachycardia Syndrome (POTS) to maintain energy levels and support overall health. Here are three nutritious and filling recipes for protein-packed sandwiches and wraps:

1. Turkey and Avocado Wrap:

Ingredients:

- 1 large whole grain or gluten-free wrap
- 3 oz sliced turkey breast
- 1/4 avocado, sliced
- Handful of spinach leaves
- 1/4 cup shredded carrots
- 1 tablespoon hummus or Greek yogurt spread
- Salt and pepper to taste

Instructions:

- Lay the wrap flat on a clean surface.
- Spread hummus or Greek yogurt spread evenly over the wrap.
- Layer sliced turkey breast, avocado slices, spinach leaves, and shredded carrots on top.
- Season with salt and pepper to taste.
- Roll the wrap tightly, tucking in the sides as you go.
- Slice in half diagonally and serve.

Benefits: This wrap provides lean protein from turkey breast, healthy fats from avocado, fiber from vegetables, and complex carbohydrates from the whole grain wrap. It's balanced and satisfying for a nutritious meal.

2. Chickpea Salad Sandwich:

Ingredients:

- 1 can chickpeas, rinsed and drained

- 1/4 cup diced celery
- 1/4 cup diced red onion
- 1/4 cup diced pickles
- 1/4 cup Greek yogurt or vegan mayo
- 1 tablespoon Dijon mustard
- Salt and pepper to taste
- Whole grain bread or gluten-free bread
- Lettuce leaves or spinach

Instructions:

- In a mixing bowl, mash chickpeas with a fork until chunky.
- Add diced celery, red onion, pickles, Greek yogurt or vegan mayo, and Dijon mustard. Mix well to combine.
- Season with salt and pepper to taste.
- Toast whole grain bread slices if desired.
- Spread chickpea salad onto bread slices.
- Top with lettuce leaves or spinach.

- Close the sandwich and slice in half.
- Serve immediately or wrap for later.

Benefits: This sandwich is high in plant-based protein from chickpeas, fiber from vegetables, and provides a creamy texture with Greek yogurt or vegan mayo. It's a satisfying and hearty option.

3. Grilled Chicken and Hummus Wrap

Ingredients:

- 1 large whole grain or gluten-free wrap
- 4 oz grilled chicken breast, sliced
- 2 tablespoons hummus (flavor of your choice)
- 1/4 cup shredded lettuce
- 1/4 cup sliced cucumber
- 1/4 cup shredded carrots
- Optional: Sliced tomatoes, bell peppers

- Salt and pepper to taste

Instructions:

- Lay the wrap flat on a clean surface.
- Spread hummus evenly over the wrap.
- Layer grilled chicken breast slices, shredded lettuce, sliced cucumber, shredded carrots, and any optional vegetables.
- Season with salt and pepper to taste.
- Roll the wrap tightly, folding in the sides as you go.
- Slice in half diagonally and serve.

Benefits: This wrap offers protein from grilled chicken breast, fiber and vitamins from vegetables, and healthy fats from hummus. It's easy to customize with different hummus flavors and additional veggies.

Tips for Customization:

- **Vegetarian Option:** Substitute grilled chicken with grilled tofu or tempeh for a plant-based alternative.

- **Gluten-Free Option:** Use gluten-free wraps or lettuce leaves as a substitute for bread.

- **Additions:** Include sliced avocado, cheese (or dairy-free cheese), or a sprinkle of seeds (such as sunflower seeds) for added flavor and nutrition.

These protein-packed sandwiches and wraps are versatile and can be adjusted based on personal preferences and dietary needs. They provide a balanced combination of protein, carbohydrates, healthy fats, and essential nutrients to support energy levels and overall well-being for individuals managing POTS. Adjust ingredients as needed and consult with a healthcare provider or dietitian for personalized dietary recommendations.

Electrolyte-Rich Soups Recipes

Electrolyte-rich soups can be beneficial for individuals with Postural Orthostatic Tachycardia Syndrome (POTS) to help maintain hydration and electrolyte balance. Here are three nutritious and flavorful soup recipes that are rich in electrolytes:

1. Chicken and Vegetable Soup:

Ingredients:

- 1 tablespoon olive oil
- 1 onion, diced
- 2 cloves garlic, minced
- 2 carrots, diced
- 2 celery stalks, diced
- 1 zucchini, diced
- 6 cups low-sodium chicken or vegetable broth
- 2 cups cooked shredded chicken breast
- 1 cup cooked quinoa or brown rice

- Salt and pepper to taste
- Fresh parsley or cilantro, chopped (for garnish)

Instructions:

- Heat olive oil in a large pot over medium heat.
- Add diced onion and minced garlic. Cook until softened and fragrant, about 3-4 minutes.
- Add diced carrots, celery, and zucchini. Cook for another 5 minutes until vegetables start to soften.
- Pour in chicken or vegetable broth and bring to a boil.
- Reduce heat to low and simmer for 15-20 minutes, until vegetables are tender.
- Stir in shredded chicken and cooked quinoa or brown rice.
- Season with salt and pepper to taste.

- Ladle soup into bowls and garnish with chopped parsley or cilantro.
- Serve hot and enjoy the electrolyte-rich soup.

Benefits: This soup is packed with electrolytes from the broth, potassium from vegetables like carrots and celery, and protein from chicken and quinoa or brown rice. It's comforting and nourishing for POTS management.

2. Coconut-Lime Vegetable Soup

Ingredients:

- 1 tablespoon coconut oil
- 1 onion, diced
- 2 cloves garlic, minced
- 1 bell pepper (any color), diced
- 1 sweet potato, peeled and diced
- 1 can coconut milk (full-fat for creaminess)

- 4 cups low-sodium vegetable broth
- Juice and zest of 1 lime
- Salt and pepper to taste
- Fresh cilantro, chopped (for garnish)

Instructions:

- Heat coconut oil in a large pot over medium heat.
- Add diced onion and minced garlic. Cook until softened and translucent, about 3-4 minutes.
- Add diced bell pepper and sweet potato. Cook for another 5 minutes, stirring occasionally.
- Pour in coconut milk and vegetable broth. Bring to a simmer.
- Cover and cook for 15-20 minutes, until sweet potatoes are tender.
- Stir in lime juice and zest. Season with salt and pepper to taste.

- Ladle soup into bowls and garnish with chopped fresh cilantro.
- Serve hot and enjoy the electrolyte-rich soup.

Benefits: This soup is rich in electrolytes from coconut milk, potassium from sweet potatoes, and vitamin C from bell peppers and lime. It's creamy, tangy, and satisfying for a nourishing meal.

3. Lentil and Spinach Soup:

Ingredients:

- 1 tablespoon olive oil
- 1 onion, diced
- 2 carrots, diced
- 2 celery stalks, diced
- 2 cloves garlic, minced
- 1 cup dried green or brown lentils, rinsed
- 6 cups low-sodium vegetable broth

- 1 teaspoon ground cumin
- 1 teaspoon ground turmeric
- Salt and pepper to taste
- 2 cups fresh spinach leaves
- Fresh parsley, chopped (for garnish)

Instructions:

- Heat olive oil in a large pot over medium heat.
- Add diced onion, carrots, and celery. Cook until softened, about 5-7 minutes.
- Add minced garlic, dried lentils, ground cumin, and ground turmeric. Cook for another minute until fragrant.
- Pour in vegetable broth and bring to a boil.
- Reduce heat to low, cover, and simmer for 20-25 minutes, until lentils are tender.

- Stir in fresh spinach leaves and cook for 2-3 minutes until wilted.
- Season with salt and pepper to taste.
- Ladle soup into bowls and garnish with chopped fresh parsley.
- Serve hot and enjoy the electrolyte-rich soup.

Benefits: This soup provides electrolytes from vegetable broth, iron and folate from lentils, and vitamins from spinach. It's hearty, wholesome, and perfect for maintaining hydration and energy levels.

Tips for Customization:

• **Protein Boost:** Add cooked chicken, tofu, or beans to any of these soups for additional protein.

• **Grains:** Experiment with adding quinoa, brown rice, or barley for added texture and nutrients.

• **Spices:** Adjust the seasoning with your favorite herbs and spices to suit your taste preferences.

These electrolyte-rich soup recipes are versatile and can be adapted based on personal preferences and dietary needs. They provide a nourishing option for individuals managing POTS, helping to maintain hydration and support overall well-being.

Adjust ingredients as needed and consult with a healthcare provider or dietitian for personalized dietary recommendations.

CHAPTER EIGHT
Balanced And Satisfying Main Courses Recipes For Dinner

Creating balanced and satisfying main courses is essential for individuals managing Postural Orthostatic Tachycardia Syndrome (POTS). These recipes are designed to provide a good balance of protein, carbohydrates, healthy fats, and nutrients to support energy levels and overall well-being.

1. Baked Salmon with Quinoa and Roasted Vegetables:

Ingredients:

- 4 salmon fillets
- 1 cup quinoa, rinsed
- 2 cups low-sodium vegetable broth or water
- 1 bunch asparagus, trimmed
- 1 bell pepper (any color), sliced
- 1 zucchini, sliced

- 2 tablespoons olive oil
- 2 cloves garlic, minced
- 1 lemon, sliced
- Salt and pepper to taste
- Fresh herbs (such as dill or parsley), chopped for garnish

Instructions:

- Preheat oven to 400°F (200°C).
- In a saucepan, bring vegetable broth or water to a boil. Add quinoa, reduce heat to low, cover, and simmer for 15-20 minutes until quinoa is cooked and liquid is absorbed.
- Meanwhile, arrange salmon fillets on a baking sheet lined with parchment paper. Season with salt, pepper, and minced garlic. Place lemon slices on top of each fillet.
- Toss asparagus, bell pepper, and zucchini with olive oil, salt, and

pepper. Spread them around the salmon on the baking sheet.
- Bake in the preheated oven for 15-20 minutes, or until salmon is cooked through and vegetables are tender.
- Fluff quinoa with a fork and divide onto plates. Top with baked salmon fillets and roasted vegetables.
- Garnish with chopped fresh herbs.
- Serve hot and enjoy this balanced and satisfying main course.

Benefits: This dish is rich in omega-3 fatty acids from salmon, protein from both salmon and quinoa, fiber from quinoa and vegetables, and vitamins from fresh herbs and vegetables.

2. Quinoa Stuffed Bell Peppers:

Ingredients:

- 4 bell peppers (any color), tops removed and seeded

- 1 cup quinoa, rinsed
- 2 cups low-sodium vegetable broth or water
- 1 tablespoon olive oil
- 1 onion, diced
- 2 cloves garlic, minced
- 1 can black beans, rinsed and drained
- 1 cup corn kernels (fresh or frozen)
- 1 teaspoon ground cumin
- 1 teaspoon chili powder
- Salt and pepper to taste
- 1/2 cup shredded cheese or dairy-free alternative (optional)
- Fresh cilantro, chopped for garnish

Instructions:

- Preheat oven to 375°F (190°C).
- In a saucepan, bring vegetable broth or water to a boil. Add quinoa, reduce heat to low, cover, and simmer for 15-

20 minutes until quinoa is cooked and liquid is absorbed.
- Heat olive oil in a large skillet over medium heat. Add diced onion and cook until softened, about 5 minutes.
- Add minced garlic, black beans, corn kernels, ground cumin, and chili powder to the skillet. Cook for another 2-3 minutes until heated through.
- Stir in cooked quinoa and mix well. Season with salt and pepper to taste.
- Stuff each bell pepper with the quinoa mixture and place them upright in a baking dish.
- If using cheese, sprinkle it over the stuffed bell peppers.
- Cover with foil and bake in the preheated oven for 25-30 minutes, until peppers are tender.
- Garnish with chopped fresh cilantro before serving.

- Serve hot and enjoy this nutritious and satisfying main course.

Benefits: These stuffed bell peppers are packed with protein from quinoa and black beans, fiber from vegetables and quinoa, and essential nutrients. They can be customized with additional toppings or spices according to personal preferences.

3. Stir-Fried Tofu and Vegetable Quinoa Bowl

Ingredients:

- 1 cup quinoa, rinsed
- 2 cups low-sodium vegetable broth or water
- 1 tablespoon sesame oil
- 1 block firm tofu, cubed
- 1 bell pepper (any color), sliced
- 1 cup broccoli florets
- 1 carrot, julienned

- 2 tablespoons soy sauce or tamari (gluten-free option)
- 1 tablespoon rice vinegar
- 1 tablespoon honey or maple syrup
- 2 cloves garlic, minced
- 1 teaspoon grated ginger
- Salt and pepper to taste
- Sesame seeds for garnish

Instructions:

- In a saucepan, bring vegetable broth or water to a boil. Add quinoa, reduce heat to low, cover, and simmer for 15-20 minutes until quinoa is cooked and liquid is absorbed.
- Heat sesame oil in a large skillet or wok over medium-high heat. Add cubed tofu and cook until golden brown on all sides, about 5-7 minutes. Remove tofu from skillet and set aside.

- In the same skillet, add bell pepper, broccoli florets, and julienned carrot. Stir-fry for 3-4 minutes until vegetables are tender-crisp.
- In a small bowl, whisk together soy sauce or tamari, rice vinegar, honey or maple syrup, minced garlic, and grated ginger.
- Return tofu to the skillet and pour the sauce over the tofu and vegetables. Stir well to coat evenly.
- Season with salt and pepper to taste.
- Divide cooked quinoa into bowls and top with stir-fried tofu and vegetables.
- Garnish with sesame seeds before serving.
- Serve hot and enjoy this flavorful and balanced main course.

Benefits: This stir-fry bowl provides protein from tofu, fiber from quinoa and vegetables, and healthy fats from sesame oil. It's packed with flavors and nutrients, making it a satisfying meal option.

Tips for Customization:

- **Add Greens:** Include spinach, kale, or arugula to any of these dishes for an extra boost of vitamins and minerals.

- **Nuts and Seeds:** Sprinkle with toasted nuts (such as almonds or cashews) or seeds (such as sunflower or pumpkin seeds) for added texture and nutrients.

- **Sauces and Dressings:** Experiment with different sauces or dressings to vary flavors, such as tahini sauce, pesto, or salsa.

These balanced and satisfying main course recipes provide a variety of nutrients essential for managing POTS symptoms while offering delicious flavors and textures. Adjust ingredients based on personal preferences and consult with a healthcare provider or dietitian for personalized dietary recommendations.

Easy And Quick Dinner Ideas Recipes

Here are three easy and quick dinner ideas that are nutritious and suitable for individuals managing Postural Orthostatic Tachycardia Syndrome (POTS). These recipes focus on simplicity and balanced nutrition:

1. One-Pan Lemon Herb Chicken with Roasted Vegetables:

Ingredients:

- 4 boneless, skinless chicken breasts
- 1 pound baby potatoes, halved
- 1 bunch asparagus, trimmed
- 1 lemon, sliced
- 3 tablespoons olive oil
- 2 cloves garlic, minced
- 1 teaspoon dried thyme (or herb of choice)
- Salt and pepper to taste
- Fresh parsley, chopped for garnish

Instructions:

- Preheat oven to 400°F (200°C).
- Place chicken breasts in the center of a large baking sheet lined with parchment paper.
- Arrange halved baby potatoes and trimmed asparagus around the chicken.
- Drizzle olive oil over chicken and vegetables. Sprinkle minced garlic, dried thyme, salt, and pepper evenly.
- Place lemon slices on top of each chicken breast.
- Bake in the preheated oven for 20-25 minutes, or until chicken is cooked through and vegetables are tender.
- Garnish with chopped fresh parsley before serving.
- Serve hot and enjoy this easy and flavorful dinner.

Benefits: This one-pan meal provides protein from chicken, carbohydrates from potatoes, fiber and vitamins from asparagus, and citrusy flavor from lemon. It's a balanced and satisfying option that requires minimal preparation.

2. Mediterranean Chickpea Salad:

Ingredients:

- 1 can chickpeas, rinsed and drained
- 1 cucumber, diced
- 1 bell pepper (any color), diced
- 1 cup cherry tomatoes, halved
- 1/4 cup red onion, thinly sliced
- 1/4 cup Kalamata olives, sliced
- 1/4 cup crumbled feta cheese or dairy-free alternative
- Juice of 1 lemon
- 3 tablespoons extra virgin olive oil
- 1 teaspoon dried oregano
- Salt and pepper to taste

- Fresh parsley, chopped for garnish

Instructions:

- In a large bowl, combine chickpeas, diced cucumber, diced bell pepper, cherry tomatoes, red onion, Kalamata olives, and crumbled feta cheese.
- In a small bowl or jar, whisk together lemon juice, extra virgin olive oil, dried oregano, salt, and pepper.
- Pour the dressing over the salad ingredients and toss gently to combine.
- Garnish with chopped fresh parsley.
- Serve immediately as a refreshing and nutritious dinner option.

Benefits: This Mediterranean-inspired salad is rich in plant-based protein from chickpeas, fiber from vegetables, healthy fats from olive oil and olives, and calcium from feta cheese. It's quick to prepare and packed with flavors.

3. Veggie Stir-Fry with Tofu and Brown Rice:

Ingredients:

- 1 block firm tofu, cubed
- 1 tablespoon sesame oil
- 1 bell pepper (any color), sliced
- 1 cup broccoli florets
- 1 carrot, julienned
- 1 cup snap peas or snow peas
- 2 cloves garlic, minced
- 2 tablespoons soy sauce or tamari (gluten-free option)
- 1 tablespoon rice vinegar
- 1 tablespoon honey or maple syrup
- 1 teaspoon grated ginger
- Cooked brown rice, for serving
- Sesame seeds for garnish

Instructions:

- Heat sesame oil in a large skillet or wok over medium-high heat.
- Add cubed tofu and cook until golden brown on all sides, about 5-7 minutes. Remove tofu from skillet and set aside.
- In the same skillet, add sliced bell pepper, broccoli florets, julienned carrot, and snap peas or snow peas. Stir-fry for 3-4 minutes until vegetables are tender-crisp.
- Add minced garlic and grated ginger to the skillet. Cook for another minute until fragrant.
- In a small bowl, whisk together soy sauce or tamari, rice vinegar, honey or maple syrup.
- Return tofu to the skillet and pour the sauce over the tofu and vegetables. Stir well to coat evenly.
- Serve stir-fry over cooked brown rice.

- Garnish with sesame seeds before serving.
- Enjoy this quick and nutritious dinner.

Benefits: This veggie stir-fry provides protein from tofu, fiber and vitamins from vegetables, and complex carbohydrates from brown rice. It's a balanced and satisfying meal that can be customized with your favorite vegetables and sauces.

Tips for Customization:

- **Protein Variations:** Substitute chicken, shrimp, or tempeh for tofu in stir-fry recipes.

- **Grain Options:** Swap brown rice with quinoa, couscous, or noodles.

- **Additions:** Include additional herbs, spices, or nuts for extra flavor and texture.

These easy and quick dinner ideas are nutritious, delicious, and designed to support individuals managing POTS with balanced meals that provide essential nutrients. Adjust ingredients based on personal preferences and dietary needs.

Slow Cooker And One-Pot Meals Recipes

Slow cooker and one-pot meals are excellent options for individuals managing Postural Orthostatic Tachycardia Syndrome (POTS) because they require minimal preparation and can be left to cook without constant monitoring. Here are three comforting and easy recipes:

1. Slow Cooker Chicken and Vegetable Stew:

Ingredients:

- 4 boneless, skinless chicken thighs
- 4 cups low-sodium chicken broth
- 1 onion, diced
- 2 carrots, sliced
- 2 celery stalks, sliced

- 1 cup baby potatoes, halved
- 1 cup green beans, trimmed and halved
- 2 cloves garlic, minced
- 1 teaspoon dried thyme
- Salt and pepper to taste
- Fresh parsley, chopped for garnish

Instructions:

- Place chicken thighs in the slow cooker.
- Add diced onion, sliced carrots, sliced celery, halved baby potatoes, and trimmed green beans.
- Pour chicken broth over the ingredients in the slow cooker.
- Add minced garlic, dried thyme, salt, and pepper.
- Stir gently to combine.
- Cover and cook on low for 6-8 hours or on high for 3-4 hours, until chicken

is cooked through and vegetables are tender.
- Remove chicken thighs from the slow cooker and shred with two forks.
- Return shredded chicken to the slow cooker and mix well.
- Adjust seasoning if needed.
- Serve hot, garnished with chopped fresh parsley.

Benefits: This hearty stew is rich in protein from chicken thighs, vitamins and fiber from vegetables, and comforting flavors from herbs. It's easy to prepare and provides a complete meal in one pot.

2. One-Pot Lentil and Vegetable Curry

Ingredients:

- 1 cup dried green or brown lentils, rinsed
- 4 cups low-sodium vegetable broth

- 1 onion, diced
- 2 cloves garlic, minced
- 1 bell pepper (any color), diced
- 1 zucchini, diced
- 1 carrot, diced
- 1 can coconut milk (full-fat for creaminess)
- 2 tablespoons curry powder
- 1 teaspoon ground turmeric
- Salt and pepper to taste
- Fresh cilantro, chopped for garnish

Instructions:

- In a large pot or Dutch oven, combine rinsed lentils, vegetable broth, diced onion, minced garlic, diced bell pepper, diced zucchini, and diced carrot.
- Bring to a boil over medium-high heat.

- Reduce heat to low, cover, and simmer for 20-25 minutes, until lentils and vegetables are tender.
- Stir in coconut milk, curry powder, ground turmeric, salt, and pepper.
- Simmer for an additional 5-10 minutes to allow flavors to meld.
- Adjust seasoning if needed.
- Serve hot, garnished with chopped fresh cilantro.
- Enjoy this flavorful and nutritious curry.

Benefits: This one-pot curry provides plant-based protein from lentils, vitamins and fiber from vegetables, and healthy fats from coconut milk. It's warming, satisfying, and can be customized with additional spices or vegetables.

3. Slow Cooker Beef and Vegetable Chili:

Ingredients:

- 1 pound lean ground beef (or ground turkey or chicken)
- 1 onion, diced
- 2 cloves garlic, minced
- 1 bell pepper (any color), diced
- 1 zucchini, diced
- 1 can (15 oz) kidney beans, rinsed and drained
- 1 can (15 oz) black beans, rinsed and drained
- 1 can (15 oz) diced tomatoes
- 1 cup low-sodium beef or vegetable broth
- 2 tablespoons chili powder
- 1 teaspoon ground cumin
- Salt and pepper to taste

- Optional toppings: shredded cheese, chopped green onions, sour cream or Greek yogurt

Instructions:

- In a skillet, cook ground beef over medium heat until browned. Drain excess fat if needed.
- Transfer cooked beef to the slow cooker.
- Add diced onion, minced garlic, diced bell pepper, diced zucchini, kidney beans, black beans, diced tomatoes (with juices), beef or vegetable broth, chili powder, ground cumin, salt, and pepper to the slow cooker.
- Stir to combine all ingredients.
- Cover and cook on low for 6-8 hours or on high for 3-4 hours.
- Adjust seasoning if needed before serving.

- Ladle chili into bowls and top with optional toppings such as shredded cheese, chopped green onions, or sour cream/Greek yogurt.
- Enjoy this hearty and flavorful chili.

Benefits: This slow cooker chili is packed with protein from ground beef and beans, fiber from vegetables and beans, and warming spices. It's a comforting meal that can be easily customized with different toppings.

Tips for Customization:

- **Vegetarian/Vegan Options:** Substitute meat with tofu, tempeh, or additional beans in recipes.

- **Spice Level:** Adjust the amount of spices and seasonings based on personal preference.

- **Additions:** Incorporate extra vegetables or grains like quinoa into these dishes for added nutrition and texture.

These slow cooker and one-pot meal recipes are convenient, nutritious, and perfect for individuals managing POTS who need easy-to-prepare meals that provide balanced nutrition.

Adjust ingredients based on dietary preferences and consult with a healthcare provider or dietitian for personalized recommendations.

CHAPTER NINE
Healthy Snack Options Recipes

Here are three healthy snack options that are convenient, nutritious, and suitable for individuals managing Postural Orthostatic Tachycardia Syndrome (POTS):

1. Greek Yogurt Parfait with Berries and Nuts

Ingredients:

- 1 cup plain Greek yogurt (or dairy-free alternative)
- 1/2 cup mixed berries (such as strawberries, blueberries, raspberries)
- 1/4 cup granola (choose low-sugar and gluten-free if needed)
- 2 tablespoons chopped nuts (such as almonds, walnuts, or pecans)
- Drizzle of honey or maple syrup (optional)

Instructions:

- In a bowl or glass, layer Greek yogurt, mixed berries, and granola.
- Sprinkle chopped nuts on top.
- Drizzle with honey or maple syrup for added sweetness if desired.
- Serve immediately and enjoy this protein-rich and nutrient-dense snack.

Benefits: This parfait provides protein from Greek yogurt, antioxidants and fiber from berries, healthy fats and crunch from nuts, and energy-sustaining carbohydrates from granola. It's balanced and satisfying for a quick snack.

2. Veggie Sticks with Hummus

Ingredients:

- Assorted vegetable sticks (such as carrots, cucumbers, bell peppers, celery)

- 1/4 cup hummus (choose your favorite flavor)

Instructions:

- Wash and cut assorted vegetables into sticks.
- Serve with hummus for dipping.
- Enjoy this crunchy and nutrient-packed snack.

Benefits: This snack is low in calories but high in fiber, vitamins, and minerals from vegetables, and provides plant-based protein and healthy fats from hummus. It's refreshing and helps maintain energy levels.

3. Energy Bites

Ingredients:

- 1 cup rolled oats (gluten-free if needed)

- 1/2 cup nut butter (such as almond butter or peanut butter)
- 1/4 cup honey or maple syrup
- 1/4 cup ground flaxseed or chia seeds
- 1/2 cup mini chocolate chips or dried fruit (optional)
- 1 teaspoon vanilla extract
- Pinch of salt

Instructions:

- In a large bowl, combine rolled oats, nut butter, honey or maple syrup, ground flaxseed or chia seeds, chocolate chips or dried fruit (if using), vanilla extract, and salt.
- Stir until well combined and mixture holds together.
- Roll mixture into bite-sized balls using your hands.
- Place energy bites on a baking sheet lined with parchment paper.

- Chill in the refrigerator for at least 30 minutes to firm up.
- Store in an airtight container in the refrigerator for up to one week.
- Enjoy these homemade energy bites as a quick and satisfying snack.

Benefits: These energy bites are packed with fiber from oats and flaxseed/chia seeds, protein and healthy fats from nut butter, and natural sweetness from honey or maple syrup. They're portable and great for a quick energy boost.

Tips for Customization:

- **Allergy-Friendly:** Adjust recipes to accommodate allergies or dietary restrictions, such as using dairy-free yogurt or nut-free alternatives.

- **Add Varieties:** Incorporate different fruits, seeds, or spices to personalize flavors and textures.

- **Portion Control:** Pre-portion snacks into small containers or bags for easy grab-and-go options.

These healthy snack options are designed to provide sustained energy, essential nutrients, and convenience for individuals managing POTS. They're easy to prepare and can be adapted to suit personal taste preferences and dietary needs.

Hydrating Beverages Recipes

Staying hydrated is crucial for individuals managing Postural Orthostatic Tachycardia Syndrome (POTS). Here are three hydrating beverage recipes that are refreshing, nutritious, and supportive of hydration:

1. Citrus Electrolyte Drink

Ingredients:

- 2 cups coconut water (unsweetened)
- Juice of 1 lemon
- Juice of 1 lime
- 1-2 tablespoons honey or maple syrup (optional for sweetness)
- Pinch of sea salt

Instructions:

- In a pitcher, combine coconut water, lemon juice, lime juice, and honey or maple syrup (if using).
- Stir until well mixed.
- Add a pinch of sea salt and stir again.
- Chill in the refrigerator before serving, or serve over ice.
- Enjoy this hydrating and electrolyte-rich beverage.

Benefits: This drink provides electrolytes from coconut water, vitamin C from citrus fruits, and optional natural sweetness from honey or maple syrup. It helps replenish electrolytes lost through sweating and supports hydration.

2. Cucumber Mint Infused Water

Ingredients:

- 1/2 cucumber, thinly sliced
- 1/4 cup fresh mint leaves
- 1 lemon, thinly sliced
- 6 cups water

Instructions:

- In a large pitcher, combine cucumber slices, fresh mint leaves, and lemon slices.
- Fill the pitcher with water.
- Refrigerate for at least 1 hour (or overnight) to allow flavors to infuse.
- Serve chilled over ice.

- Enjoy this refreshing and hydrating infused water.

Benefits: This infused water is hydrating and provides a refreshing flavor from cucumber, mint, and lemon. It's a great alternative to plain water and encourages increased fluid intake.

3. Watermelon Coconut Water Slushie

Ingredients:

- 2 cups seedless watermelon, cubed
- 1 cup coconut water (unsweetened)
- Juice of 1 lime
- Ice cubes

Instructions:

- In a blender, combine cubed watermelon, coconut water, and lime juice.
- Add a handful of ice cubes.

- Blend until smooth and slushie-like consistency.
- Pour into glasses and serve immediately.
- Enjoy this hydrating and refreshing slushie.

Benefits: This slushie is hydrating with electrolytes from coconut water and provides hydration and vitamins from watermelon and lime. It's a delicious way to cool down and stay hydrated.

Tips for Customization:

• **Herb Infusions:** Experiment with different herbs like basil or rosemary in infused water for varied flavors.

• **Fruit Varieties:** Substitute watermelon with other fruits like berries, pineapple, or oranges in slushie recipes.

- **Sweeteners:** Adjust sweetness levels in drinks based on personal preference or dietary needs.

These hydrating beverage recipes are easy to prepare and can be enjoyed throughout the day to support hydration and overall well-being for individuals managing POTS. Adjust ingredients based on taste preferences and consult with a healthcare provider or dietitian for personalized hydration recommendations.

Salt-Rich Snacks Recipes

For individuals managing Postural Orthostatic Tachycardia Syndrome (POTS), it's important to maintain adequate salt intake to help manage symptoms like low blood pressure and orthostatic intolerance. Here are three salt-rich snack recipes that can help increase salt intake in a nutritious way:

1. Homemade Trail Mix

Ingredients:

- 1 cup mixed nuts (such as almonds, cashews, peanuts)
- 1/2 cup pumpkin seeds
- 1/2 cup sunflower seeds
- 1/2 cup dried cranberries or raisins
- 1/2 teaspoon sea salt (adjust to taste)
- Optional: 1/4 cup dark chocolate chips or chunks

Instructions:

- In a large bowl, combine mixed nuts, pumpkin seeds, sunflower seeds, dried cranberries or raisins, and sea salt.
- Add dark chocolate chips or chunks if desired for a touch of sweetness and additional flavor.
- Toss well to mix all ingredients evenly.
- Store in an airtight container or portion into small snack bags.

- Enjoy this salt-rich trail mix as a convenient snack option.

Benefits: This homemade trail mix provides a combination of healthy fats, protein, fiber, and essential minerals from nuts and seeds. The added sea salt enhances the salt content, making it a suitable snack to increase sodium intake.

2. Avocado Toast with Sea Salt

Ingredients:

- 2 slices whole grain bread (gluten-free if needed), toasted
- 1 ripe avocado, mashed
- Sea salt, to taste
- Optional toppings: cherry tomatoes, cucumber slices, red pepper flakes

Instructions:

- Toast whole grain bread slices until golden brown.
- Spread mashed avocado evenly on each slice of toast.
- Sprinkle sea salt generously over the avocado.
- Add optional toppings such as cherry tomatoes, cucumber slices, or red pepper flakes for extra flavor and texture.

- Serve immediately and enjoy this simple and salt-rich snack.

Benefits: Avocado provides healthy fats, fiber, and potassium, while sea salt enhances the sodium content. Whole grain bread adds complex carbohydrates for sustained energy.

3. Salted Edamame

Ingredients:

- 2 cups frozen edamame (in pods or shelled)
- Sea salt, to taste

Instructions:

- Cook frozen edamame according to package instructions (boil in salted water for about 5 minutes if in pods).
- Drain and pat dry with paper towels.
- Sprinkle sea salt over the cooked edamame while still warm.

- Toss to coat evenly with salt.
- Serve warm or at room temperature.
- Enjoy this quick and nutritious salt-rich snack.

Benefits: Edamame is a good source of plant-based protein, fiber, and essential minerals. Sea salt adds sodium content to help increase salt intake beneficial for individuals with POTS.

Tips for Customization:

- **Spice Variations:** Add spices like chili powder, paprika, or garlic powder to trail mix or avocado toast for added flavor.

- **Nutritional Yeast:** Sprinkle nutritional yeast over edamame for a cheesy flavor boost along with salt.

- **Portion Control:** Pre-portion snacks into small containers or bags for easy grab-and-go options throughout the day.

These salt-rich snack recipes provide options for increasing sodium intake in a balanced and nutritious way, supporting individuals managing POTS in maintaining hydration and managing symptoms effectively. Adjust salt levels according to personal preference and consult with a healthcare provider or dietitian for personalized dietary recommendations.

CHAPTER TEN
Exercise And Physical Activity

Exercise and physical activity can play a crucial role in managing Postural Orthostatic Tachycardia Syndrome (POTS) by improving cardiovascular fitness, enhancing blood circulation, and increasing overall strength and stamina. Here are some key considerations and recommendations for individuals with POTS:

1. Types of Exercise:

a. Aerobic Exercise:

- **Low-Intensity Cardio:** Start with activities like walking, stationary cycling, or swimming at a gentle pace. Gradually increase duration and intensity as tolerated.

- **Interval Training:** Alternating short bursts of higher intensity with periods of rest can help improve cardiovascular fitness without excessive strain.

b. Strength Training:

• **Bodyweight Exercises:** Include exercises like squats, lunges, push-ups, and planks to build muscle strength and endurance.

• **Light Weights or Resistance Bands:** Incorporate resistance training to strengthen muscles without causing excessive fatigue.

c. Flexibility and Balance Exercises:

• **Yoga or Pilates:** These exercises focus on flexibility, balance, and core strength, which can help improve posture and stability.

• **Stretching:** Gentle stretching exercises can help prevent muscle stiffness and improve overall flexibility.

2. Exercise Guidelines:

- **Start Slowly:** Begin with short sessions of exercise and gradually increase duration and intensity over time.

- **Listen to Your Body:** Pay attention to symptoms such as dizziness, lightheadedness, or palpitations. Rest as needed and avoid pushing beyond your limits.

- **Hydration and Electrolytes:** Drink plenty of fluids and consider increasing salt intake before and after exercise to help maintain hydration and prevent symptoms.

- **Cooling Measures:** Stay cool during exercise to avoid overheating, such as using fans, wearing breathable clothing, and exercising in air-conditioned environments.

3. Exercise Modifications:

- **Vertical Exercises:** Individuals with POTS may benefit from exercises performed in a reclined or seated position to minimize orthostatic stress.

- **Pacing:** Break exercise into shorter sessions throughout the day rather than one prolonged session to manage symptoms effectively.

- **Postural Changes:** Gradually incorporate changes in posture (e.g., from sitting to standing) to improve tolerance over time.

4. Monitoring Progress:

- **Keep Track:** Maintain a journal to track exercise sessions, symptoms, and any changes in tolerance or improvement in fitness over time.

- **Consult with Healthcare Providers:** Work closely with healthcare providers, including cardiologists, physiotherapists, or exercise physiologists, to develop an individualized exercise plan.

5. Safety Precautions:

• **Avoid Overexertion:** Balance exercise with adequate rest and recovery periods to prevent exacerbation of symptoms.

• **Seek Guidance:** If symptoms worsen or new symptoms arise during exercise, consult with a healthcare provider promptly for guidance.

Example Exercise Plan:

• **Warm-up:** 5-10 minutes of gentle stretching or walking.

• **Aerobic Exercise:** 20-30 minutes of low-impact cardio (e.g., walking on a treadmill or cycling).

• **Strength Training:** 10-15 minutes of bodyweight exercises (e.g., squats, push-ups) or light resistance exercises.

- **Cool-down:** 5-10 minutes of stretching or relaxation exercises.

Adjust the intensity and duration of each exercise based on individual tolerance and progress. Consistency is key to reaping the benefits of exercise while managing symptoms effectively. Always prioritize safety and listen to your body's signals during physical activity.

Managing Stress And Sleep

Managing stress and ensuring adequate sleep are essential components of managing Postural Orthostatic Tachycardia Syndrome (POTS) effectively. Here are some strategies and recommendations for coping with stress and improving sleep quality:

Managing Stress:

Mindfulness and Relaxation Techniques:

- **Deep Breathing:** Practice diaphragmatic breathing or paced breathing exercises to calm the nervous system and reduce stress.

- **Meditation:** Incorporate mindfulness meditation or guided relaxation sessions to promote relaxation and mental clarity.

- **Progressive Muscle Relaxation:** Practice tensing and relaxing different muscle groups to release tension and promote relaxation.

Physical Activity:

- Engage in regular physical activity such as yoga, tai chi, or gentle stretching exercises to reduce stress and improve overall well-being.

- Exercise releases endorphins, which can help elevate mood and reduce stress levels.

Healthy Lifestyle Habits:

- Maintain a balanced diet with regular meals and adequate hydration.

- Limit caffeine and alcohol intake, as they can exacerbate stress and interfere with sleep.

- Ensure regular and balanced meals to stabilize blood sugar levels, which can affect mood and stress levels.

Social Support:

- Connect with friends, family, or support groups to share experiences and receive emotional support.

- Talking to others who understand your condition can provide comfort and reduce feelings of isolation.

Time Management and Prioritization:

- Break tasks into manageable steps and prioritize responsibilities to avoid feeling overwhelmed.
- Set realistic goals and expectations for yourself, recognizing that some days may require more rest and self-care than others.

Improving Sleep Quality:

Establish a Sleep Routine:

- Maintain a consistent sleep schedule by going to bed and waking up at the same time each day, even on weekends.

- Create a calming bedtime routine, such as reading a book, taking a warm bath, or practicing relaxation techniques before bed.

Create a Comfortable Sleep Environment:

- Ensure your bedroom is conducive to sleep by keeping it cool, dark, and quiet.

- Use comfortable bedding and pillows that support your body and promote relaxation.

Limit Stimulants Before Bed:

- Avoid caffeine and nicotine in the hours leading up to bedtime, as they can interfere with sleep.

- Limit screen time (e.g., phones, computers, TVs) before bed to reduce exposure to blue light, which can disrupt sleep patterns.

Manage Stress and Anxiety:

- Practice stress-reducing techniques (mentioned above) to calm the mind and prepare for sleep.

- Consider journaling or writing down worries before bed to help clear your mind.

Address Sleep Disorders:

- If you suspect a sleep disorder (e.g., insomnia, sleep apnea), consult with a healthcare provider for evaluation and treatment options.

Additional Tips:

- **Hydration:** Ensure adequate hydration throughout the day, but reduce fluid intake closer to bedtime to minimize disruptions from nocturia (nighttime urination).

- **Medication Management:** Discuss medications with your healthcare provider to ensure they do not interfere with sleep or exacerbate POTS symptoms.

Work with healthcare providers, including psychologists, counselors, or sleep specialists, to develop a personalized plan for managing stress and improving sleep quality.

By implementing these strategies and making lifestyle adjustments, individuals with POTS can better manage stress, improve sleep quality, and enhance overall well-being. Consistency and patience are key as you develop and refine your personalized stress management and sleep improvement plan.

CHAPTER ELEVEN
Monitoring And Adjusting Your Diet

Monitoring and adjusting your diet is crucial for managing Postural Orthostatic Tachycardia Syndrome (POTS) effectively. Here are some key steps and considerations to help you monitor and optimize your diet:

1. Keeping a Food Diary:

- **Purpose:** Start by keeping a detailed food diary to track your daily intake, including meals, snacks, beverages, and portion sizes.

- **Symptom Tracking:** Record any symptoms you experience throughout the day, such as dizziness, fatigue, or changes in heart rate.

- **Identifying Triggers:** Look for patterns between your diet and symptoms to identify potential triggers or foods that may exacerbate POTS symptoms.

2. Key Dietary Considerations:

- **Fluid and Salt Intake:** Adequate hydration and increased salt intake are often recommended for individuals with POTS to help maintain blood volume and manage symptoms.

- **Hydration:** Aim to drink plenty of fluids throughout the day, including water, herbal teas, and hydrating beverages (as discussed earlier).

- **Salt:** Consult with your healthcare provider or dietitian to determine the appropriate amount of salt (sodium) intake for your individual needs.

- **Balanced Nutrition:** Focus on a balanced diet that includes a variety of nutrient-dense foods:

- **Fruits and Vegetables:** Aim for a colorful variety to ensure a range of vitamins, minerals, and antioxidants.

- **Protein Sources:** Include lean meats, poultry, fish, eggs, legumes, nuts, and seeds for adequate protein intake.

- **Whole Grains:** Choose whole grains such as brown rice, quinoa, oats, and whole wheat bread for fiber and sustained energy.

- **Meal Timing and Frequency:** Eating smaller, more frequent meals throughout the day can help maintain stable blood sugar levels and prevent symptoms associated with postprandial hypotension (low blood pressure after eating).

3. Adjusting Your Diet:

- **Work with a Dietitian:** Consider consulting with a registered dietitian who specializes in POTS or cardiovascular health to develop a personalized nutrition plan.

- **Gradual Changes:** Make dietary adjustments gradually to observe how your body responds and to avoid overwhelming changes.

- **Elimination Diet:** If specific food triggers are suspected (e.g., gluten, dairy, certain additives), consider an elimination diet under the guidance of a healthcare professional to identify problematic foods.

4. Monitoring Progress:

- **Review Your Food Diary:** Regularly review your food diary and symptom log to assess progress and identify areas for improvement.

- **Symptom Management:** Notice any changes in symptoms based on dietary adjustments and discuss them with your healthcare team.

5. Additional Tips:

- **Educate Yourself:** Stay informed about POTS and its dietary implications through reputable sources and healthcare professionals.

- **Peer Support:** Consider joining support groups or online communities where individuals with POTS share experiences and tips on managing diet and symptoms.

- **Self-Care:** Incorporate stress management techniques and adequate sleep to support overall well-being and symptom management.

Example Diet Adjustments:

- **Increasing Salt Intake:** Incorporate salt-rich snacks (as previously discussed), add salt to meals, or choose higher-sodium options when appropriate.

- **Balancing Carbohydrates:** Opt for complex carbohydrates that provide sustained energy and avoid large meals that may trigger symptoms.

- **Managing Fluid Intake:** Monitor fluid intake to maintain hydration without exacerbating symptoms like nocturia.

By actively monitoring your diet, making informed adjustments, and collaborating with healthcare professionals, you can better manage POTS symptoms and improve overall quality of life. Personalize your approach based on individual needs and responses, aiming for a balanced and nourishing diet that supports your health goals.

Conclusion

managing Postural Orthostatic Tachycardia Syndrome (POTS) involves a multifaceted approach that includes lifestyle modifications, dietary adjustments, exercise, stress management, and adequate sleep. Individuals with POTS often experience a range of symptoms related to orthostatic intolerance and cardiovascular dysregulation, making it essential to tailor interventions to their specific needs.

Key Strategies for Managing POTS:

- **Dietary Adjustments:** Monitor salt and fluid intake, maintain balanced nutrition, and track food triggers to manage symptoms effectively.

- **Exercise and Physical Activity:** Incorporate low-impact aerobic exercises, strength training, and flexibility exercises to improve cardiovascular fitness and overall strength.

- **Stress Management:** Practice relaxation techniques, mindfulness, and ensure adequate social support to reduce stress levels and improve overall well-being.

- **Sleep Hygiene:** Establish a consistent sleep routine, create a conducive sleep environment, and address any sleep disorders to optimize sleep quality.

- **Regular Monitoring:** Keep a food diary, track symptoms, and consult healthcare professionals regularly to adjust treatment plans as needed.

Work closely with healthcare providers, including cardiologists, dietitians, and exercise physiologists, to develop a personalized management plan tailored to your specific symptoms and health goals. Stay informed about POTS through reliable sources and connect with support groups or online communities to learn from others' experiences and share strategies.

A thorough strategy that takes into account both mental and physical health is necessary for the management of POTS, as is perseverance and patience. Individuals suffering from POTS can ameliorate their symptoms, raise their quality of life, and improve their health in general by following the methods described and gradually adjusting to them.

Always put yourself first, speak up for what you need, and consult with medical experts; your POTS path will be different from everyone else's, so take care of yourself. Managing POTS efficiently and living a fulfilling life is achievable with determination and help.

THE END

www.ingramcontent.com/pod-product-compliance
Lightning Source LLC
Chambersburg PA
CBHW071829210526
45479CB00001B/47